Easy Copyca

CW00458509

365 Days of Easy and Tasty Recipes.
Enjoy the Best Mouth-watering Dishes and
Move the First Steps into the Kitchen with The
Most Famous Chipotle, Olive Garden,
Applebee's Recipes.

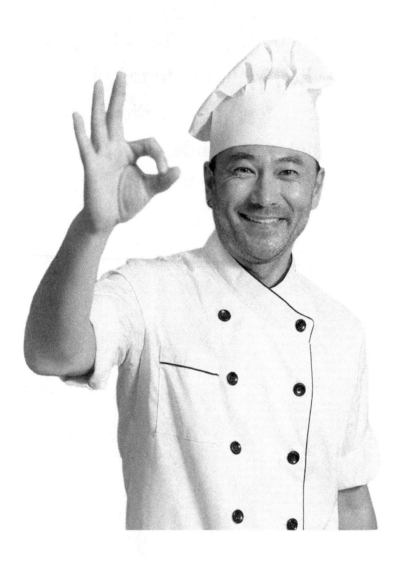

TABLE OF CONTENTS

INTRODUCTION

Recipes use basic ingredients that can be found in any grocery store. It is not really that hard to study how to cook top-secret eatery recipes. Some contemplate you need a cooking education or degree in culinary arts so you can cook those secret recipes. I hate telling you this, but anybody can gather the fixings themselves then cook an extravagant meal that palates similar the real thing.

Copycat restaurant recipes are now widely known because of the ever-high cost of eating out. These copycat restaurant recipes are the hidden recipes from all your favorite restaurants in America so you can prepare them in the comfort of your home.

The benefit of using copycat restaurant recipes is that not only can you save money; you can also customize the recipes. For example, if you want to decrease the butter or salt in one of the plates, you can. Now you've kept money, and at the same time providing a nourishing meal for your family.

You have little control over the ingredients in the meal when you eat out. You can't, of course, adjust the dish that you order because sauces, etc. are made in advance. All of us know that it is expensive to take our family out for dinner, and without a doubt, this would easily cost you around a hundred dollars on an average. With copycat restaurant recipes the same one hundred dollars can easily produce 4 or more meals. Having consistent meals enthused by your preferred restaurants as a family permits for a healthier, extra tight-knit family. Study have shown that, families who dine together at home are more united, and the kids perform better.

Cooking recipes copied from restaurants will also amaze your friends and family who will ask

themselves "where did you learn to cook so well?". Imagine cooking a whole meal that appears to be the restaurant's takeaway food. I bet some of your friends won't even believe you cooked it! Regular low-cost meals will always be more appreciated than irregular expensive meals. Your family's

favorite restaurant recipes and specials are the result of both skills and hard work of talented chefs. It is just a matter of going through the steps to get the same results.

The basic information you need to make restaurant recipes is similar whether you are cooking French or Italian dishes. The secret dishes made by professional chefs, are the result of careful study, experience and practice. You can learn a great deal from them and become a better cook.

Creating similar meals just takes time and knowledge of the basics. It may be said that creating a meal at home is very easy, but when you try to do or experiment it by yourself, it costs both time and money. Try to remember that there is always a substitution you can make in many of these recipes because home cooking allows for the creativity of brilliant young chefs who don't always go

by the traditional recipe book.

BREAKFAST RECIPES

California Kitchen Pizza ® Italian Chopped Salad

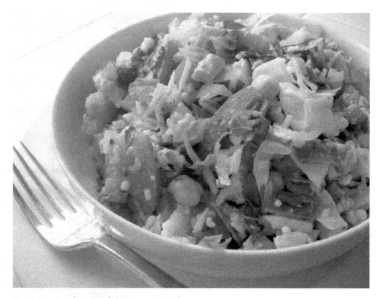

Preparation Time: 30 minutes

Cooking Time: 0 minutes

Servings: 6

Ingredients:

Mixed greens:

- 1 big head (4 cups; 285g) romaine lettuce
- 1 can (15 oz.; 439g) chickpeas (additionally called garbanzo grains), drained pipes and washed
- 1 pint (2 cups; 300g) antique cherry tomatoes cut into quarters

- 1/2 cup (48g) extremely thinly cut reddish onion
- 1 cup (4 oz.; 120g) chopped salami
- 1/2 cup (80g) chopped pork
- 1 cup (5oz, 140g) fresh mozzarella gems, halved
- 1/3 cup (40g) thinly sliced pepperoncini
- 10-12 sizable fresh basil leaves behind

Dressing:

- 2 tablespoons freshly pressed lemon extract
- 2 tablespoons Dijon mustard
- 3 tablespoons cabernet white vinegar
- 3 teaspoons white colored sweets
- 1 tsp dried oregano
- 1 tsp dried out parsley
- 1 clove garlic (1/2 tsp lessened)
- 1/3 cup olive oil
- Sodium and pepper

Directions:

Dressing:

1. Place every one of the dressing ingredients in a wide-mouth container. Season with salt and pepper— I add 1/2 teaspoon salt, and 1/4 teaspoon pepper. Place the bottle cover, and quickly shake to blend. Sure, place bottle in the refrigerator and outlet there until all set to dress the salad that was tossed.

Lettuce:

2. Wash and cut the lettuce. I like to reduce the salad into ribbons (wrap the items right into stogies and afterwards

very finely slice) and after that halve the ribbons--thinner mixed greens parts allow additional surface for the dressing to stick to. Utilize a mixed greens rewriter to ensure the lettuce is 100% dry before including every other ingredient.

Tossed Salad Ingredients:

3. Add in the drained pipes and washed chickpeas, quartered cherry tomatoes, very finely cut reddish onion, thinly sliced salami, chopped ham, halved mozzarella gems, and very finely sliced pepperoncini.

4. Chiffonade the basil pieces (find Note 2) and add those right into the tossed salad. Toss the mixed greens and adjust add-ins to personal desire. (The amounts noted are basic tips of how we like this chopped salad. The ideal component of creating this homemade is you can easily add added garnishes to individual preference!).

Add Dressing:

5. Cut the dressing from the refrigerator and drink for recombination again. Just apply the dressing to the amount of salad you'll be immediately delighting in. The mixed greens do not fit effectively with dressing so keep it separate until it's ready to eat right away!

Surplus Dressing:

You may not utilize all the dressing in this tossed salad (outfit to desire). Leftover dressing maintains to a week in the fridge.

Nutrition: Calories 313; Carbs 24g; Protein 48g; Fat 82g

Cheddar ® Honey Butter Croissants

Preparation Time: 40 minutes

Cooking Time: 25 minutes

Servings: 12

Ingredients:

- Croissant Dough:
- 3 1/2 cup all-purpose flour plus more to flour work surface
- 1 1/3 cup milk
- 2 1/4 tsp yeast (1 envelope)
- 1 1/2 tsp salt
- 2 tbsp. vegetable oil
- 1 tbsp. granulated sugar
- 1 1/2 cup butter cold, 3 sticks
- Egg Wash
- 1 egg
- 1 tsp heavy whipping cream
- Honey Butter Drizzle:
- 1/4 cup unsalted butter
- 2 1/2 tbsp. honey
- 3 tbsp. powdered sugar

Directions:

For the Croissant Dough:

1. Combine flour, milk, yeast, salt, vegetable oil, and sugar using a stand mixer with a dough hook. Mix the dough on low for 3 minutes. If you do not have a stand mixer,

mix the ingredients together with a spoon until they begin to thicken, then kneed it with your hands. The dough is ready when it no longer is so sticky that it clings to your fingers or the dough hook. Dough should be tacky, but easy to detach and roll into a ball.

2. Grease a large bowl with butter, and then place the croissant dough ball inside. Cover bowl with plastic wrap and allow dough to rise for 1-2 hours in a warm environment. Tip: I ran my dryer on low heat for 20 minutes, turned it off, and then placed the bowl inside with the door closed.

3. While dough rises, cut each stick of cold butter lengthwise into 3 pieces. Place butter slices in a Ziploc bag (quart sized), arranging them in as close to a flat layer as possible. Using a rolling pin, roll and press the butter so that the edges fuse together and the butter reaches the edges of the bag. This will create a solid 8x8 square of butter. Cut butter out of Ziploc bag, and then wrap the butter square in plastic wrap. Place butter back in the refrigerator until dough is ready.

4. Once dough has risen, the next step is to "laminate" the dough, which is a special technique of folding the cold butter within the croissant dough. Once dough has been laminated, refrigerate it overnight. Remove cold dough from refrigerator. Prepare 2 baking sheets by lining them with parchment paper. Dough must remain cold while working (to prevent butter within from melting), so before beginning, divide the dough in half. Keep one

half to work with and place the other half in the refrigerator so that it remains cold until ready to be used.

5. Generously flour your work space. Place dough down and roll into a 7 x 20" rectangle, using more flour to prevent sticking as necessary. Cut triangles within the dough, making the small point about 1/4 inch wide and the wide end about 4-5 inches wide. Once cut, roll croissants starting from the wide base toward the small point. Place croissants on the baking sheet 2 inches apart. If desired, curl the ends of the croissant for a more decorative look. Remove the other half of the dough from the refrigerator and repeat the same steps.

6. Prepare egg wash by whisking together egg and cream. Coat croissants generously with egg wash using a pastry brush.

7. Allow croissants to rise for another 1-3 hours at room temperature. Dough will puff slightly and should wiggle if baking dish is lightly shaken. Preheat oven to 375 F. Bake croissants for 25-35 minutes or until tops are golden brown.

For the Honey Butter Drizzle:

8. In a microwave safe bowl, heat butter until melted, about 45 seconds. Whisk in honey and powdered sugar. If the honey will not fully dissolve, heat the sauce for another 20 seconds.

Putting It All Together:

9. Serve croissants warm with honey butter drizzled on top or as a dipping sauce on the side.

Nutrition: Calories 440; Fat 30g; Carbs 36g; Protein 5g

Panera Bread® Caramel Pecan Rolls

Preparation Time: 15 minutes

Cooking Time: 25 minutes

Servings: 2-4

Ingredients:

- 1 cup of milk
- 1/4 cup water
- 1/4 cup sugar
- 1/4 cup butter
- 1/6 cup cornmeal
- 1 teaspoon salt
- 3 1/2 cups all-purpose flour
- 1 package (1/4 oz.) active dry yeast
- 1 large egg

Topping

- 1 cup packed brown sugar
- 1/4 cup butter
- 1/4 cup milk
- 1/2 cup pecans, chopped

Filling

- 1/8 cup butter, softened
- 1/4 cup sugar
- 1 teaspoon ground cinnamon

Directions:

1. Take a suitable-sized saucepan and place it over medium-high heat. Add milk, water, sugar, butter,

cornmeal, and salt to the saucepan. Stir cook this cornmeal mixture to a boil, then remove it from the heat and allow it to cool. Meanwhile, mix 2 cups flour with yeast in a mixing bowl;

2. Beat the cornmeal mixture in a mixing bowl on low speed until smooth. Add flour mixture to the cornmeal and mix well until smooth. Stir in 1 cup flour, and eggs then whisk well until it makes soft dough. Transfer this cornmeal dough to a lightly floured surface and knead it for 8 minutes;

3. Grease glass bowl with cooking oil and place the dough in the bowl. Cover the cornmeal dough with a plastic sheet and leave it for 1 hour at a warm place in the kitchen. Meanwhile, prepare the topping by mixing sugar, butter, and milk in a small bowl. Pour this topping into a greased 8 inches baking pan and drizzle pecans on top;

4. Remove the flour dough from the bowl and divide it into two halves. Roll each dough piece into 8X5 inches rectangle. Top each rectangle with butter and then drizzle cinnamon and sugar over this layer. Now roll each dough sheet from its long side and pinch the seams to seal. Slice each roll into 4 slices to get a shape of a pinwheel. Place these cinnamon rolls in the prepared pan, layered with topping mixture;

5. Cover the cinnamon rolls with a kitchen towel and leave them for 30 minutes. Now bake the cinnamon rolls for 25 minutes in the oven at 375 degrees F. Once baked,

remove the cinnamon rolls pan from the oven and leave it for 1 minute. Flip the pan over a plate and remove it from the top. Serve the cinnamon rolls.

Nutrition: Calories 720, Carbs 69g, Fat 46g; Protein 11g

IHOP® Tilapia Florentine

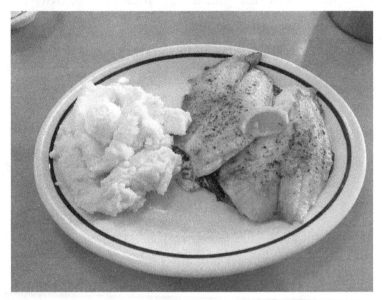

Preparation Time: 30 minutes

Cooking Time: 20 minutes

Servings: 4

Ingredients:

- 1 package (6 ounces) fresh baby spinach
- 6 teaspoons canola oil, divided
- 4 tilapia fillets (4 ounces each)
- 1 egg, lightly beaten
- 2 tablespoons lime juice
- 2 teaspoons garlic-herb seasoning blend
- 1/4 cup grated Parmesan cheese
- 1/2 cup part-skim ricotta cheese

Directions:

1. Cook the spinach in 4 teaspoons of oil until wilted in a large non-stick skillet; drain. In the meantime, put tilapia in a fattened 13-in. x in Baking platter. Drizzle with remaining lime juice and oil. Sprinkle with a blend to season.
2. Combine the egg, ricotta cheese and spinach in a small bowl; spoon filets over. Sprinkle with a cheese made with Parmesan. Bake for 15-20 minutes at 375 °, or quickly with a fork until the fish flakes.

Nutrition: Calories 680; Fat 43g; Carbs 34g; Protein 43g

IHOP ® Original Buttermilk Pancake

Preparation Time: 10 minutes

Cooking Time: 10 minutes

Servings: 8

Ingredients:

- 1 1/4 cups sifted all-purpose flour
- 1 teaspoon baking powder
- 1 teaspoon baking soda
- 1 large egg, beaten
- 1 1/4 cups buttermilk
- 1/8 Teaspoon salt
- 3 Tablespoons sugar
- 2 Tablespoons butter, melted

Directions:

1. Firstly, put the flour, baking powder, baking soda and salt together in a big pot. Combine egg and buttermilk in a medium saucepan. Whisk in before mixing. Add mixture to the rice, stirring until smooth. Add the melted butter and sugar to whisk and bake until mixed.

2. Place on medium-low heat a griddle or non-stick skillet— grease griddle with spray or butter to cook. Drop one-fourth cup batter into the pan and spread into a circle of 5 inches. Cook until surface bubbles begin to form, and edges start to brown. Flip softly to the other hand and switch to brown. Repeat with batter left over. Serve with simmering butter and sweet syrup.

Nutrition: Calories 670; Fat 24g; Carbs 94g; Protein 4g

IHOP® Crepe

Preparation Time: 10 minutes

Cooking Time: 20 minutes

Servings: 4

Ingredients:

- 1 cup all-purpose flour
- 2 eggs
- 1/2 cup milk
- 1/4 teaspoon salt
- 1/2 cup water
- 2 tablespoon melted butter

Directions:

1. Mix the flour and eggs in a bowl until combined. Add milk and water and then mix again until evenly combined. Finally, finish off the batter with butter and salt applied. Keep whisking until the batter gets smooth.

2. Heat a non-stick saucepan and add the butter. When the butter has heated a little, ladle some of the batter over it. Spread the batter slightly by tilting the pan, and cook the bottom side until golden brown. Now turn the crepe onto the other side to get the same color. Make this way all the crepes, and serve soft.

Nutrition: Calories 1120; Fat 75g: Carbs 52g: Protein 60g

MAIN RECIPES

Chicken Alfredo

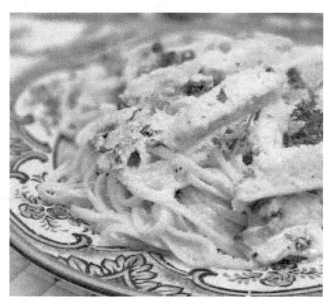

Preparation Time: 10 minutes

Cooking Time: 10 minutes

Servings: 4

Ingredients

- ¾ pound fettuccine pasta
- 2 tablespoons olive oil
- ½ cup + 2 tablespoons butter (divided)
- 2 boneless skinless chicken breasts
- 1½ teaspoons salt (divided)
- 1½ teaspoons fresh ground pepper (divided)
- 3 cloves garlic, very finely chopped

- 1½ tablespoons flour
- 2 cups heavy cream
- ¾ cup grated parmesan
- 2 tablespoons parsley

Directions

1. Cook pasta according to package instructions. Drain and set aside. Cook oil in a cast iron grill pan over high heat. Add 2 tablespoons of butter to the pan and then add the chicken breasts. Season the chicken breasts well.

2. Cook the first side until golden brown. Flip, cover the pan, and reduce the heat to medium. Cook until the chicken is cooked thoroughly. Set aside and cover in foil. Once cooled, cut into strips.

3. Cook remaining butter over medium heat in a big, deep skillet. Add garlic and cook for about 30 seconds. Reduce to medium-low heat and season with remaining salt and pepper. Add flour, whisking constantly to break up any chunks. Slowly pour the cream into the mixture. Cook until sauce is slightly thickened.

4. Stir in the parmesan until smooth. Remove from heat and set aside. Serve by tossing the pasta with the alfredo sauce. Place chicken on top and garnish with fresh parsley and parmesan, if desired.

Nutrition: 431 calories 6g carbohydrates 35g protein

Parmesan Crusted Chicken

Preparation Time: 15 minutes
Cooking Time: 40 minutes
Servings: 4

Ingredients

Breading

- 1 cup plain breadcrumbs
- 2 tablespoons flour
- ¼ cup grated parmesan cheese

For dipping

- 1 cup milk

Chicken

- 2 chicken breasts
- Vegetable oil for frying
- 2 cups cooked linguini pasta
- 2 tablespoons butter
- 3 tablespoons olive oil
- 2 teaspoons crushed garlic
- ½ cup white wine
- ¼ cup water
- 2 tablespoons flour
- ¾ cup half-and-half
- ¼ cup sour cream
- ½ teaspoon salt
- 1 teaspoon fresh flat leave parsley, finely diced¾ cup mild Asiago cheese, finely grated

Garnish

- 1 Roma tomato, diced
- Grated parmesan cheese
- Fresh flat leaf parsley, finely chopped

Directions

1. Pound the chicken until it flattens to ½ inch thick. Mix the breading ingredients in one shallow bowl and place the milk in another. Heat some oil over medium to medium-to-low heat.
2. Dip the chicken in the breading, then the milk, then the breading again. immediately place into the heated oil. Cook the chicken in the oil until golden brown, about 3-4 minutes per side. Remove the chicken and set aside on a plate lined with paper towels.
3. Create a roux by adding flour to heated olive oil and butter over medium heat. When the roux is done, add the garlic, water, and salt to the pan and stir. Add the wine and continue stirring and cooking.
4. Add the half-and-half and sour cream and stir some more. Add the cheese and let it melt. Finally, add in the parsley and remove from heat. Add pasta and stir to coat.
5. Divide the hot pasta between serving plates. Top each dish with the chicken, diced tomatoes, and parmesan cheese before serving.

Nutrition: 481 calories 7.6g carbohydrates 31g protein

Chicken Giardino

Preparation Time: 10 minutes

Cooking Time: 20 minutes

Servings: 4

Ingredients

Sauce

- 1 tablespoon butter
- ¼ teaspoon dried thyme
- ½ teaspoon fresh rosemary, finely chopped
- 1 teaspoon garlic pepper seasoning
- 1 tablespoon cornstarch
- ¼ cup chicken broth
- ¼ cup water
- ¼ cup white wine
- 1 tablespoon milk
- 1 teaspoon lemon juice
- Salt and pepper

Chicken

- 2 pounds boneless skinless chicken breasts
- ¼ cup extra virgin olive oil
- 2 small rosemary sprigs
- 1 clove garlic, finely minced
- Juice of ½ lemon

Vegetables

- ¼ cup extra-virgin olive oil

- ½ bunch fresh asparagus (remove bottom inch of stem, cut remainder into 1-inch pieces)
- 1 zucchini, julienned
- 1 summer squash, julienned
- 2 roma tomatoes, cut into ½-inch pieces
- ½ red bell pepper, julienned
- 1 cup broccoli florets, blanched
- ½ cup frozen peas
- 1 cup spinach, cut into ½-inch pieces
- ½ cup carrot, julienned
- 1-pound farfalle pasta (bow ties)

Directions

1. Using a saucepan, cook butter over medium heat. Add the thyme, garlic, pepper, and rosemary. Whisk together and cook for 1 minute. In a mixing bowl, mix together the chicken broth, water, wine, milk, and lemon juice. Slowly pour in the cornstarch and whisk constantly until it has dissolved.
2. Pour the mixture into the saucepan. Whisk well and then bring to a boil. Season with salt and pepper to taste, then remove from heat.
3. Prepare the chicken by cutting into strips width-wise. In a mixing bowl, combine the olive oil, rosemary, garlic, and lemon juice. Marinate the chicken for 30 minutes.
4. Heat ¼ cup of olive oil over medium-high heat in a saucepan. Cook the chicken strips until internal temperature is 165°F. Add the vegetables to the saucepan and sauté until cooked. Prepare the pasta according to

package instructions. Drain. Add the pasta and pasta sauce to the sauté pan.

5. Toss to thoroughly coat pasta and chicken in sauce. Serve.

Nutrition: 481 calories 6.5g carbohydrates 30g protein

Chicken and Sausage Mixed Grill

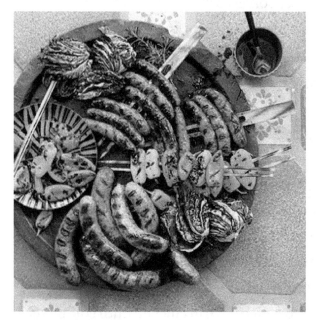

Preparation Time: 10 minutes

Cooking Time: 35 minutes

Servings: 4

Ingredients

Marinade

- 2 teaspoons red pepper oil
- 2 tablespoons fresh rosemary, chopped
- ½ cup fresh lemon juice
- 1 teaspoon salt
- 3 bay leaves, broken into pieces
- 2 large garlic cloves, pressed
- ¼ cup extra-virgin olive oil
- Freshly shredded parmesan cheese, for serving

Skewers

- 3 lemons
- 2 pounds skinless, boneless chicken breasts
- 1-pound Italian sausage links, mild
- 1-pint cherry tomatoes
- 2 rosemary sprigs

Directions

1. To make the marinade, mix pepper oil, rosemary, lemon juice, salt, bay leaves and pressed garlic in a baking dish. Cut the chicken breasts in half lengthwise. Pierce each chicken piece with a skewer and thread through. Add a cherry tomato at the end of the skewer. Coat each skewer with the marinade. Chill for at least 3 hours.

2. Prep oven to 350°F. Bake sausage for 20 minutes. Let cool, then cut into 3 pieces. Grill chicken until completely cooked. Place sausages on skewers. Grill. Serve by garnishing with rosemary, lemon, and cherry tomatoes on a platter. Sprinkle with freshly shredded parmesan, if desired.

Nutrition: 469 calories 7g carbohydrates 32g protein

Chicken Gnocchi Veronese

Preparation Time: 20 minutes

Cooking Time: 25 minutes

Servings: 4

Ingredients

- ¼ cup extra-virgin olive oil
- 1 small Vidalia onion, chopped
- 1 red bell pepper, julienned
- ½ zucchini, julienned
- Salt to taste
- 4 chicken breasts, sliced in ½-inch strips
- 2 small sprigs rosemary
- 1 glove garlic, minced
- Juice of ½ lemon

Veronese Sauce

- 1 cup parmesan cheese, grated
- ½ cup ricotta cheese
- 14 ounces heavy cream

Gnocchi

- 2 quarts water
- 1 1/3cups all-purpose flour
- 2 eggs
- 2 pounds russet potatoes
- 2 teaspoons salt or 1-pound gnocchi (potato dumplings), cooked according to package directions

Directions

1. If using pre-made gnocchi, cook according to package instructions. If not, begin by washing potatoes and placing them in water. Cook potatoes until soft. Remove water and cool in the refrigerator. Once cooled, peel and push potatoes through a fine grater or rice grater.

2. Incorporate potatoes and eggs. Slowly add flour until the dough does not stick to your hands. Divide dough into four. Roll each section into a long rope. Cut into ½-inch pieces, then create impressions by gently pushing a fork into the gnocchi.

3. Fill in water into a pot and bring to a boil. Add gnocchi and cook until they begin to float. Using a mixing bowl, stir in the garlic, lemon juice, rosemary, and chicken slices. Marinate for 2 hours. In another bowl, mix the parmesan cheese, ricotta cheese, and heavy cream.

4. Heat the olive oil in a sauté pan over medium-high heat. Add the onion, bell peppers and zucchini. Sauté until the onion is translucent. Situate chicken to the sauté pan and cook until brown. Reduce heat and add the sauce. Simmer. Mix in gnocchi and toss to coat in the sauce. Serve with additional parmesan cheese, if desired.

Nutrition: 521 calories 5.9g carbohydrates 31g protein

Chicken Parmigiana

Preparation Time: 20 minutes
Cooking Time: 25 minutes
Servings: 4

Ingredients

- 4 boneless, skinless chicken breasts (½ pound each)
- 2 cups flour
- ½ quart milk
- 4 eggs
- 3 cups Italian breadcrumbs
- ½ cup marinara sauce
- 1 cup mozzarella cheese
- ½ cup vegetable oil
- Parsley (to garnish)
- Cooked pasta with marinara sauce to serve

Directions

1. Put flour in a bowl. In another bowl, mix milk and eggs together. In a third bowl, place breadcrumbs. Place chicken breasts between plastic wrap and pound to about ¼ inch in thickness. Season with salt and pepper.
2. Place chicken in flour, coating all sides. Dip into egg wash then bread crumbs, coating each side evenly. Preheat oven to broil. In a cast iron pan, heat oil over medium heat. Fry both side of the chicken for 10 minutes. Drain on paper towels.
3. Place chicken on a baking dish. Top with marinara sauce and mozzarella cheese. Place in oven until cheese is melted. Garnish with parsley. Serve with a side of marinara pasta, if desired.

Nutrition: 489 calories 6.7g carbohydrates 34g protein

Chicken and Shrimp Carbonara

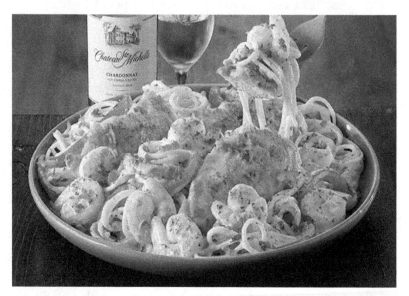

Preparation Time: 35 minutes

Cooking Time: 40 minutes

Servings: 8

Ingredients

Shrimp Marinade

- ¼ cup extra virgin olive oil
- ½ cup water
- 2 teaspoons Italian seasoning
- 1 tablespoon minced garlic

Chicken

- 4 boneless and skinless chicken breasts cubed
- 1 egg mixed with 1 tablespoon cold water
- ½ cup panko bread crumbs
- ½ cup all-purpose flour
- ½ teaspoon salt

- ½ teaspoon black pepper
- 2 tablespoons olive oil

Carbonara sauce

- ½ cup butter (1 stick)
- 3 tablespoons all-purpose flour
- ½ cup parmesan cheese, grated
- 2 cups heavy cream
- 2 cups milk
- 8 Canadian bacon slices, diced finely
- ¾ cup roasted red peppers, diced

Pasta

- 1 teaspoon salt
- 14 ounces spaghetti or bucatini pasta (1 package)
- Water to cook the pasta

Shrimp

- ½ pound fresh medium shrimp, deveined and peeled
- 1-2 tablespoons olive oil for cooking

Direction

1. Incorporate all the marinade ingredients together in a re-sealable container or bag and add the shrimp. Refrigerate for at least 30 minutes.
2. To make the chicken, mix the flour, salt, pepper, and panko bread crumbs into a shallow dish. Scourge egg with 1 tablespoon of cold water in a second shallow dish. Dip the chicken into the breadcrumb mix and after in the egg wash, and again in the breadcrumb mix. Place on a plate and let rest until all the chicken is prepared.

3. Warm the olive oil over medium heat in a deep large skillet. Working in batches, add the chicken. Cook for 12 minutes on both sides. Situate the cooked chicken tenders on a plate lined with paper towels to absorb excess oil.

4. To make the pasta, add water to a large pot and bring to a boil. Sprinkle salt and cook the pasta according to package instructions about 10-15 minutes before the sauce is ready.

5. To make the shrimp, while the pasta is cooking, add olive oil to a skillet. Remove the shrimp from the marinate and shake off the excess marinade. Cook the shrimp for 2-3 minutes.

6. To make the Carbonara sauce, in a large deep skillet, sauté the Canadian bacon with a bit of butter for 3-4 minutes over medium heat or until the bacon starts to caramelize. Add the garlic and sauté for 1 more minute. Remove bacon and garlic and set aside.

7. In the same skillet, let the butter melt and mix-in the flour. Slowly stir in the cream and milk and whisk until the sauce thickens. Add the cheese.

8. Decrease the heat to a simmer and keep the mixture simmering while you prepare the rest of the ingredients.

9. Mix in drained pasta, bacon bits, roasted red peppers to the sauce. Stir to coat. Add pasta evenly to each serving plate. Top with some chicken and shrimp. Garnish with fresh parsley Serve with fresh shredded Romano or Parmesan cheese

Nutrition: 488 calories 6.7g carbohydrates 33g proteins

Chicken Marsala

Preparation Time: 10 minutes

Cooking Time: 40 minutes

Servings: 4 - 6

Ingredients

- 2 tablespoons olive oil
- 2 tablespoons butter
- 4 boneless skinless chicken breasts
- 1 ½ cups sliced mushrooms
- 1 small clove garlic, thinly sliced
- Flour for dredging
- Sea salt and freshly ground black pepper
- 1 ½ cups chicken stock
- 1 ½ cups Marsala wine
- 1 tablespoon lemon juice
- 1 teaspoon Dijon mustard

Directions

Chicken scaloppini

1. Press down the chicken with a mallet or rolling pin to about ½ inch thick Using a big skillet, cook olive oil and 1 tablespoon of the butter over medium-high heat. When the oil is hot, dredge the chicken in flour. Season on both sides. Dredge only as many as will fit in the skillet. Don't overcrowd the pan.

2. Cook chicken in batches, about 1 to 2 minutes on each side or until cooked through. Remove from skillet, and

place on an oven-proof platter. Keep warm, in the oven, while the remaining chicken is cooking.

Marsala sauce

1. In the same skillet, pour in 1 tablespoon of olive oil. On medium-high heat, sauté mushrooms and garlic until softened. Pull out mushrooms from the pan and set aside.

2. Add the chicken stock and loosen any remaining bits in the pan. On high heat, let reduce by half, about 6-8 minutes. Add Marsala wine and lemon juice and in the same manner reduce by half, about 6–8 minutes. Add the mushroom back in the saucepan, and stir in the Dijon mustard. Warm for 1 minute on medium-low heat. Take away from heat, mix in the remaining butter to make the sauce silkier. Pour sauce over chicken, and serve.

Nutrition: 487 calories 7.1g carbohydrates 34g protein

Chicken Scampi

Preparation Time: 10 minutes
Cooking Time: 20 minutes
Servings: 4
Ingredients
Pasta

- ½ pound uncooked angel hair pasta
- ½ teaspoon canola or olive oil
- ¼ teaspoon salt

Chicken

- 1-pound chicken tenderloins
- ½ cup all-purpose flour
- ¼ teaspoon salt
- 1/8 teaspoon ground pepper
- ¼ teaspoon Italian seasoning
- 1/3 cup whole milk
- 2 tablespoons oil

Vegetables and sauce

- 2 tablespoons canola or olive oil
- ½ green pepper, sliced into thin strips
- ½ red pepper, sliced into thin strips
- ½ yellow pepper, sliced into thin strips
- ½ red onion, sliced thin
- 5 tablespoons unsalted butter
- 6 cloves garlic, minced
- ¾ cup wine

- 1 1/3 cups chicken broth
- 2/3 cup half and half
- ¼ teaspoon ground pepper
- 1 teaspoon salt
- ¼ teaspoon Italian seasoning

Directions

1. Cook the angel hair pasta following to package instructions. Drain and set aside.
2. To make the chicken, mix the flour, salt, pepper and Italian seasoning in a bowl. Place the milk in a separate bowl. Lightly pound the chicken tenders, then coat them in flour. Dip into milk and dredge in flour once more.
3. Using big skillet, cook oil over high heat. Cook each sides of the chicken for 2 minutes. Remove from heat and keep warm.
4. To make the vegetables and sauce, heat the oil in the skillet. Add the peppers and red onion. Sauté for 2 minutes over medium-high heat, stirring occasionally.
5. Add the butter and minced garlic to the vegetables. Sauté for 1 more minute. Add the wine and broth. Reduce heat to medium-low. Let cook for 5 minutes. Add half and half, salt, pepper, and Italian seasoning. Let cook for 1 minute. Add the chicken and pasta. Toss together to blend well. Simmer to warm, then serve.

Nutrition: 489 calories 6.8g carbohydrates 31g protein

Chicken Margherita

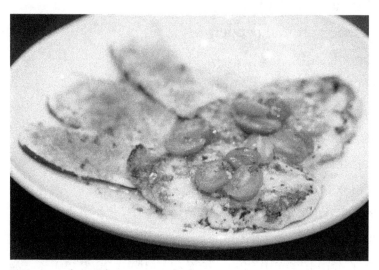

Preparation Time: 35 minutes

Cooking Time: 25 minutes

Servings: 6

Ingredients

Chicken

- 6 (4-ounce) boneless chicken breasts
- 2 cups water
- ¼ cup salt
- ¼ cup sugar

Pesto

- 2 cups fresh basil
- 1 clove garlic
- 2 tablespoons pecorino Romano cheese, grated
- 3–4 tablespoons extra-virgin olive oil
- 1 tablespoon pine nuts (optional)
- Lemon garlic sauce

- 2 tablespoons butter
- 2 cloves garlic, minced
- 1 tablespoon all-purpose flour
- 1 tablespoon lemon juice
- ½ cup low-sodium chicken broth

Chicken Margherita assembly

- 6 (4-ounce) grilled boneless chicken breasts
- ½ cup prepared pesto
- 1 cup grape tomatoes, halved
- 6 ounces fresh mozzarella, sliced
- ½ cup prepared lemon garlic sauce
- Freshly shredded parmesan cheese, for garnish

Directions

1. In a Ziploc bag, combine the water, salt, and sugar. Mix well. Add the chicken and refrigerate for at least 2 hours.
2. Grill chicken until cooked thoroughly. Set aside. Incorporate all pesto ingredients in a food processor to achieve a smooth consistency. Add 1 tablespoon of oil, if needed. Chill sealed container until ready to use.
3. To make the lemon garlic sauce, melt the butter in a small saucepan. Add garlic and sauté for 1 minute. Slowly add some flour and stir well. Add fresh lemon juice and chicken broth. Stir for about 3–5 minutes until the sauce begins to thicken. Keep refrigerated.
4. To assemble the Chicken Margherita, preheat oven to 425°F. Move the grilled chicken to a baking dish and top

with mozzarella cheese, pesto and halved grape tomatoes.

5. Pour the lemon garlic sauce on top. Bake until cheese melts, about 10–15 minutes. Drizzle with freshly grated parmesan cheese, if desired.

Nutrition: 469 calories 6.3g carbohydrates 31g protein

Chicken Carbonara

Preparation Time: 20 minutes

Cooking Time: 30 minutes

Servings: 4

Ingredients

Marinated chicken or shrimp

- 1 cup extra-virgin olive oil
- 1 cup hot water
- 1 tablespoon Italian seasoning
- 1 tablespoon chopped garlic
- 3 pounds chicken strips or large shrimp, peeled and deveined

Sauce

- 1 cup butter
- 1½ teaspoons garlic, chopped
- 3 tablespoons bacon bits
- 3 tablespoons all-purpose flour
- 1 cup parmesan cheese, grated
- 1-quart heavy cream
- 1-quart milk
- ¼ cup bacon base
- ½ teaspoon black pepper
- 1¾ pounds long pasta (spaghetti, linguine, etc.) cooked according to package directions
- ¼ teaspoon salt

Topping

- 3 tablespoons Romano cheese, grated
- 3 tablespoons parmesan cheese, grated
- 1¾ cups mozzarella cheese, shredded
- ½ cup panko breadcrumbs
- 1½ teaspoons garlic, chopped
- 1½ tablespoons butter, melted
- 2 tablespoons parsley, chopped

Marinated chicken strips (or shrimp) as above

- 1½ cups roasted red peppers
- ¼ cup bacon bits

Directions

1. Preheat oven to 350°F. Scourge olive oil with hot water, Italian seasoning and chopped garlic. Let chicken/shrimp marinate for at least 30 minutes in the refrigerator.
2. To make the sauce, melt the butter over medium heat in a large saucepan. Sauté the garlic and bacon bits for 5 minutes, stirring frequently.
3. Add the flour, parmesan cheese, heavy cream, milk, bacon base, pepper, and salt. Whisk well. Boil, then decrease heat and simmer.
4. To make the topping, mix the Romano cheese, parmesan, mozzarella cheese, panko, chopped garlic, melted butter and chopped parsley in a mixing bowl. Blend well. Set aside.
5. Heat a large skillet to cook the chicken and/or shrimp. Add the red peppers and bacon bits. Cook for 3 minutes or until meat is cooked through. Add sauce and stir.

6. Add pasta. Mix well to coat the pasta evenly. Top with extra cheese, if desired. Serve.

Nutrition: 510 calories 6.3g carbohydrates 30g protein

Steak Gorgonzola Alfredo

Preparation Time: 10 minutes

Cooking Time: 20 minutes

Servings: 6

Ingredients

- 18 ounces rib eye or sirloin steak, cut into 2–3-inch medallions
- 1-pound fettuccine
- 4 cups baby spinach
- ½ cup sun-dried tomatoes, chopped
- ½ cup gorgonzola cheese, crumbled
- Balsamic glaze (or aged balsamic), as desired

Alfredo sauce

- 3 tablespoons butter
- 3 tablespoons all-purpose flour
- 2 cups heavy cream
- ½ cup pecorino romano cheese, grated

Directions

1. First, make the alfredo sauce. Using a saucepan, cook butter over medium heat. Slowly add the flour, whisking frequently. Add the heavy cream and grated cheese. Continue to whisk until thickened.
2. Cook fettuccine according to package directions. Drain and set aside. Grill the steak to preference in a skillet. Set aside. Place the alfredo sauce in a pot and heat on low. Add the pasta and spinach. Continue to stir until the spinach wilts. Remove from heat.

3. Place the sun-dried tomatoes, gorgonzola cheese and steak on top of the pasta. Drizzle with balsamic glaze. Serve.

Nutrition: 497 calories 7.9g carbohydrates 32g protein

P.F. Chang's Crispy Honey Chicken

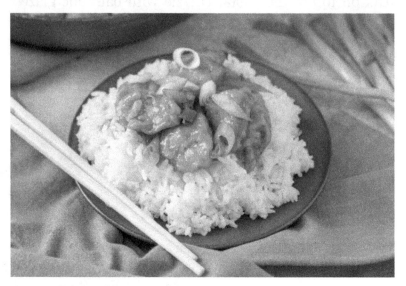

Preparation Time: 20 minutes

Cooking Time: 2 hours

Servings: 4

Ingredients

Chicken:

- 1-pound chicken breast, boneless, skinless, cut into medium sized chunks
- Vegetable oil, for frying and deep frying
- Batter:
- 4 ounces all-purpose flour
- 2½ ounces cornstarch
- 1 egg
- 6 ounces water
- 1/8 teaspoon baking powder
- 1/8 teaspoon baking soda

Chicken Seasoning:

- 1 tablespoon light soy sauce
- 1/8 teaspoon white pepper
- ¼ teaspoon kosher salt
- 1 tablespoon cornstarch

Sauce:

- ½ cup sake or rice wine
- ½ cup honey
- 3 ounces rice vinegar
- 3 tablespoons light soy sauce
- 6 tablespoons sugar
- ¼ cup cornstarch
- ¼ cup water

Directions:

1. Do the batter in advance. Combine all the batter ingredients together and refrigerate. After an hour and 40 minutes, mix all the seasoning ingredients together and mix in the chicken. Make sure that the chicken is covered entirely. Place the chicken in the refrigerator to marinate for at least 20 minutes. Except for the cornstarch and water, incorporate all the sauce ingredients together and set aside.
2. Before you begin frying your chicken:
3. Heat oil at 350 degrees. When your oil is heated, remove the chicken from the refrigerator and pour the batter all over it.

4. One by one, lower the coated chicken pieces into the heated oil. Keep them suspended until the batter is cooked (20 to 30 seconds).

5. When all the chicken is cooked, place it on the plate covered with the paper towel to cool and drain.

6. Bring the sauce mixture to a boil. While waiting to boil, incorporate cornstarch and water in a separate bowl. Slowly pour in the cornstarch mixture into the sauce and continue cooking for 2 minutes, until the sauce thickens.

7. When the sauce thickens, remove it from heat. When the chicken is cooked, pour some sauce over the entire mixture, just enough to cover the chicken. Transfer everything to a plate with rice or Chinese noodles and serve.

Nutrition: 680.3 Calories 12g Total Fat 30.7g Protein

Boston Market's Chicken Pot Pie

Preparation Time: 10 minutes

Cooking Time: 40 minutes

Serving: 4

Ingredients

- 1 cup half-and-half
- 1 cup chicken broth
- 3 tablespoons all-purpose flour
- 2 cups shredded chicken breast, roasted, skinless
- 2 cups mixed frozen vegetables, thawed
- 2 tablespoons fresh flat-leaf parsley, chopped
- 2 tablespoons chives, chopped
- 1 teaspoon fresh thyme, chopped
- 1 teaspoon lemon juice
- 1 teaspoon salt
- ½ teaspoon lemon zest, grated
- ½ teaspoon freshly ground black pepper
- 7 ounces ready-to-use refrigerated pie crust

Directions:

1. Get ready by: Preheating the oven to 425F; Lightly flouring a flat surface; and Bringing out 4 10-ounce ramekins.

2. Bring the half-and-half, broth, and flour to a boil while stirring with a whisk. Decrease heat and simmer for another 4 minutes while continuing to whisk the

mixture. When it thickens, stir in the remaining ingredients, except for the pie crust.

3. When all the ingredients are cooked, turn off the heat and cover the pan. Set the mixture aside to work on the pie crust.

4. Place the pie crust on your floured surface and roll it into a circle with an 11-inch diameter. Cut the crust into quarters. Scoop the warm chicken mixture into each of the ramekins. Cover the tops with the pie crust, letting it drape over the edges. Slice an X into each of the tops to allow the pie to cook completely. Bake the pies for 25 minutes and remove from the oven. Let rest 10 minutes before serving.

Nutrition: 450 Calories 30g Total Fat 10g Protein

PF Chang's Chicken Fried Rice

Preparation Time: 10 minutes

Cooking Time: 10 minutes

Servings: 4

Ingredients

- 2 cups prepared rice
- ½ cup frozen mixed vegetables
- 2 green onions, chopped
- 1 chicken breast seasoned with salt & pepper
- 1 clove garlic, minced
- 1 egg
- 3 teaspoons sesame or wok oil, divided
- 2 tablespoons soy sauce

Directions

1. Scourge egg and 1 teaspoon of oil. Using a wok, cook another teaspoon of the oil and cook the chicken until done. Remove from skillet and set aside.

2. Pour in last teaspoon of oil to the skillet and stir in the mixed vegetables and green onions. Cook and stir until hot and tender. Mix in garlic and cook until fragrant. Using a spatula or spoon, move the vegetables to one side. Stir in egg mixture and scramble until cooked, then add the chicken and stir until it is all combined.

Nutrition: 641 calories 9g fats 34g protein

PF Chang's Ginger Chicken with Broccoli

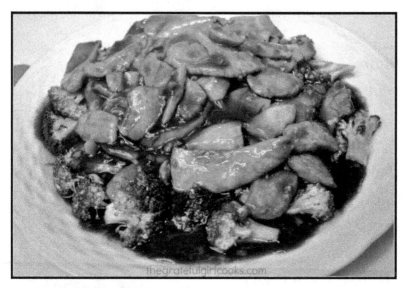

Preparation Time: 10 minutes

Cooking Time: 20 minutes

Servings: 4

Ingredients

- ½ cup egg substitute or beaten eggs
- ¼ teaspoon white pepper
- ¼ teaspoon salt
- 1-pound boneless, skinless chicken breasts, sliced

Stir-fry sauce

- ½ cup soy sauce
- 2 tablespoons rice wine vinegar
- 1 tablespoon sugar
- ½ cup chicken broth
- 3 cups chicken broth

- ½ pound broccoli florets
- 2 tablespoons butter
- 2 tablespoons ginger, freshly minced
- 2 tablespoons green onion, minced
- 1 teaspoon garlic, minced
- ¼ cup cornstarch
- 1 teaspoon sesame oil

Directions

1. In a resealable bag, combine the eggs or egg substitute, salt and pepper. Add the chicken pieces and seal. Chill for at least 3 hours. When ready to use, discard the marinade. Incorporate all of the ingredients for the stir-fry sauce in a mixing bowl. Mix well and set aside.
2. Add the 3 cups of chicken broth to a large skillet or wok and bring to a boil. Reduce heat to maintain a simmer. Stir in chicken and cook until almost done, then remove from the pot.
3. Add the broccoli to the broth and cook until tender. Then drain the broth and transfer the broccoli to a plate. Add the butter to the skillet and heat over medium heat. When melted, stir in the ginger, green onion and garlic and cook until the garlic is fragrant.
4. Return them to the skillet and cook until done, about 5 minutes.
5. Thicken the broth with a slurry made from the cornstarch and ½ cup of water. Cook until the sauce thickens. Serve the chicken over rice and broccoli.

Nutrition: 623 calories 11g fats 29g protein

Pei Wei's Spicy Chicken

Preparation Time: 10 minutes
Cooking Time: 15 minutes
Servings: 4

Ingredients

- 2 boneless skinless chicken breasts
- 1½ cups sliced carrots
- 1½ cups sugar snap peas
- 3 cups vegetable oil for frying

Batter

- 1½ cups flour
- 1½ teaspoons salt
- 1½ teaspoons baking soda
- 2 eggs
- 2/3 cup milk
- 2/3 cup water

Sauce

- 3 teaspoons vegetable oil
- 3 tablespoons minced garlic
- ¼ cup green onion, chopped, white parts only
- 1½ cups pineapple juice
- 3 teaspoons chili garlic paste, more if you want it spicier
- 3 tablespoons white wine vinegar
- 2 tablespoons sugar
- 2 teaspoons soy sauce
- 1 teaspoon salt

- 4 teaspoons cornstarch
- 3 tablespoons water

Directions

1. Incorporate all of the ingredients for the batter. It should be smooth and without lumps. It will be thinnish. Using saucepan, boil 3 cups of water then add the carrots and peas and cook just until tender. Drain and set aside.

2. Using deep fryer, cook the 3 cups of oil to 375°F. Mix in chicken to the hot oil a few pieces at a time. Leave it there until cooked through and golden brown, then transfer to a paper-towel-lined plate to drain.

3. Using a wok, cook 2 teaspoons of oil over medium-high heat. Stir in garlic and green onion and cook for about 1 minute. Mix all of the sauce ingredients except for the cornstarch and water.

4. Incorporate sauce mixture to the hot skillet and cook until it starts to bubble. Make a slurry of the cornstarch and water and add it to the bubbling sauce, and cook until the sauce starts to thicken. Add the chicken, peas and carrots and cook until hot. Serve with rice.

Nutrition: 684 calories 9g fats 31g protein

Pei Wei's Chicken Pad Thai

Preparation Time: 15 minutes

Cooking Time: 15 minutes

Servings: 4 - 6

Ingredients

- ½ cup low-fat coconut milk
- 6 tablespoons creamy peanut butter
- ¼ cup light soy sauce
- ¼ cup lime juice
- ½ tablespoon rice wine vinegar
- 2 tablespoons brown sugar
- 2 teaspoons grated ginger
- ½ teaspoon red pepper flakes

Chicken stir-fry

- ½ tablespoon canola oil
- ½ tablespoon dark sesame oil
- 1–2 teaspoons curry powder (optional)
- 1-pound chicken breast, cut into bite-sized pieces
- 6–8 ounces frozen sugar snap peas
- 1 medium onion, chopped
- 2 cloves garlic, minced
- ½ pound cooked rice noodles or long thin pasta

Garnish

- ¼ cup lightly salted dry roasted peanuts, chopped
- Cilantro

Directions

1. Incorporate all of the sauce ingredients in a mixing bowl. Combine well, then set aside. Cook the noodles following the package directions. Set aside. Cook canola oil and sesame oil in a large skillet over medium-high heat. When hot, add the chicken and stir. Cook for 5 minutes, then mix in the garlic.

2. When the chicken is completely cooked through, add the peas and cook a bit longer to heat the peas through. Stir in the sauce and make sure the chicken is evenly coated. Add the cooked noodles and stir to make sure everything is covered in the sauce. Serve with cilantro and top with chopped peanuts.

Nutrition: 612 calories 10g fats 33g protein

Pei Wei's Sesame Chicken

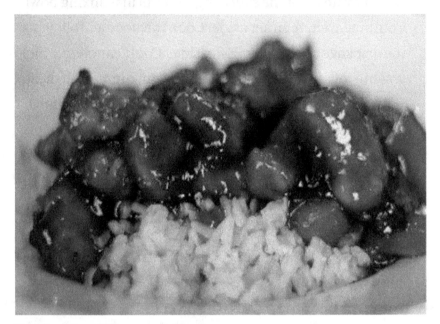

Preparation Time: 20 minutes

Cooking Time: 15 minutes

Servings: 4 - 6

Ingredients

Sauce

- ½ cup soy sauce
- 2½ tablespoons hoisin sauce
- ½ cup sugar
- ¼ cup white vinegar
- 2½ tablespoons rice wine
- 2½ tablespoons chicken broth
- Pinch of white pepper
- 1¼ tablespoons orange zest

Breaded chicken

- 2 pounds boneless skinless chicken breasts
- ¼ cup cornstarch
- ½ cup flour
- 1 egg
- 2 cups milk
- Pinch of white pepper
- Pinch of salt
- 1-quart vegetable oil
- ½ red bell pepper, chunked
- ½ white onion, chunked
- 1 tablespoon Asian chili sauce
- ½ tablespoon ginger, minced
- ¼ cup scallions, white part only, cut into rings
- 1 tablespoon sesame oil
- 1 tablespoon cornstarch
- 1 tablespoon water
- Sesame seeds for garnish

Directions

1. Prep the sauce by mixing all of the ingredients together in a small saucepan. Bring to a simmer, then remove from the heat and set aside. Scourge eggs, milk, salt and pepper together in a shallow dish.

2. Mix the ¼ cup of cornstarch and flour together in a separate shallow dish. Soak chicken pieces in the egg mixture and then in the cornstarch/flour mixture. Shake off any excess, then set aside. Cook the vegetable oil over medium-high heat in a deep skillet or saucepan.

3. When hot, drop the coated chicken into the oil and cook for about 2–4 minutes. Remove from oil and place on a paper-towel-lined plate to drain. Make a slurry out of the 1 tablespoon of cornstarch and water.

4. In a different large skillet or wok, heat 1 tablespoon of sesame oil until hot. Add the ginger and chili sauce and heat for about 10 seconds. Cook peppers and onions for another 30 seconds. Stir in the chili sauce and ginger and the sauce you made earlier and bring to a boil. Once it boils, stir in the cornstarch slurry and cook until the sauce thickens.

5. When the sauce is thick, add the chicken and stir to coat. Serve with rice, and season with sesame seeds.

Nutrition: 691 calories 10g fats 31g protein

Pei Wei's Asian Diner Caramel Chicken

Preparation Time: 20 minutes

Cooking Time: 55 minutes

Servings: 6

Ingredients

- 1 cup sugar
- ¼ cup water
- ¾ cup reduced-sodium chicken broth
- 3 tablespoons fish sauce
- 2 tablespoons soy sauce
- 1 whole chicken, cut in 10 pieces
- 1 teaspoon salt
- 2 tablespoons vegetable oil and more, if needed
- ¼ cup fresh ginger, chopped
- 2 tablespoons fresh garlic, chopped
- ½ large red onion, chopped
- 2 tablespoons jalapenos, chopped
- 1 English cucumber, sliced then julienned
- ½ red bell pepper, julienned lengthwise
- 1 carrot, cut diagonally
- 2 green onions, chopped
- ½ cup pineapple chunks
- ¼ cup fresh mint, chopped
- ¼ cup fresh cilantro, chopped
- ¼ cup fresh basil, chopped
- Cooked rice or rice vermicelli for serving

Vietnamese vinaigrette

- ½ cup lime juice, plus wedges for serving
- ¼ cup light brown sugar
- 2 tablespoons Vietnamese fish sauce
- ½ teaspoon toasted sesame oil
- 4 teaspoons vegetable oil

Directions

1. Preheat oven to 325°F. Combine sugar and water in a deep sauce pot. Bring to a boil and simmer until the sugar turns a dark caramel color.

2. Pour in chicken broth and continue stirring over low heat until the sugar dissolves. Mix in fish sauce and soy sauce. Set aside.

3. Combine the Vietnamese vinaigrette ingredients in a medium bowl and stir in cucumbers, red bell peppers and carrots. Marinate until ready to use. Season the chicken pieces with the salt.

4. Cook vegetable oil in a big Dutch oven and brown the chicken pieces on all sides. Putt aside. In the same pan, with the extra vegetable oil if needed, sauté the ginger, garlic, red onion and jalapeno at medium heat for 4–5 minutes.

5. Add the browned chicken pieces and the caramel sauce to the Dutch oven, turning the chicken in the caramel broth to coat all sides. Arrange the chicken so it is all submerged in the sauce as much as possible and boil.

6. Cover then situate in the oven and braise for 35–45 minutes. While cooking, assemble the green onion, pineapple chunks and the other herbs and set aside.

7. Sprinkle green onions and pineapple chunks and stir well. Serve the chicken over rice or rice vermicelli. Top with a portion of Vietnamese vinaigrette slaw.

Nutrition: 697 calories 12g fats 32g protein

DRESSING RECIPES

Cheese Sauce Recipe

Preparation time: 55 minutes

Cooking time: 30 minutes

Servings: 4

Ingredients

- 200 cc of cream or milk
- 80g provolone cheese
- 80g of Sardinian cheese
- 80g mozzarella cheese
- 30g blue cheese
- 500 cc of milk
- 45g butter
- 45g flour
- 1 clove garlic
- Thyme c / n
- Salt and ground black pepper c / n
- Nutmeg c / n

Direction

1. To make the sauce four kinds of cheese, place the butter in a pot and bring it to the fire.
2. Let melt and add the flour. Stir immediately with a wire whisk to make a roux and cook the pasta over the fire for a few seconds.

3. Place the milk in a saucepan together with a clove of peeled and crushed garlic and a little thyme. When it starts to boil, remove from heat and let stand covered for 15 minutes.

4. Remove the thyme and garlic clove and heat the milk again. Put it in the other pot and mix very well with some rods. Pepper to taste and add a little nutmeg. Cook for two minutes once it boils.

5. Add mozzarella, provolone cheese, Sardinian cheese or some variety of cheese with holes, and blue cheese. Bring the pot to the fire and mix with a wooden spoon so that the cheeses melt.

6. Add cream or milk cream and reserve the sauce 4 kinds of cheese.

Nutrition: 467 Calories 20g Protein 31g Fat

Copycat Chipotle Mexican Grill Spicy Corn Salsa

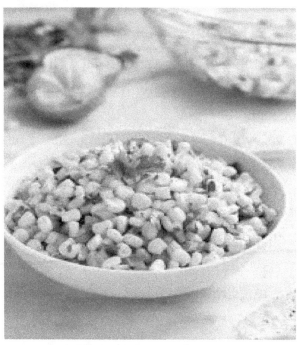

Preparation time: 21 minutes

Cooking time: 23 minutes

Servings: 4

Ingredients

- 2 cups of frozen corn
- 1/4 cup of chopped coriander
- 2 teaspoons of finely chopped jalapeno seeds removed
- 1/4 cup of chopped roasted poblano pepper
- 2 teaspoons of chopped red onions
- 1/2 teaspoon of kosher salt
- 1 teaspoon of lime juice

- 1 teaspoon of lemon juice

Direction

1. Allow frozen corn to thaw completely.
2. Preheat the oven to 425 degrees. Stir in Poblano pepper with vegetable oil. When the oven is hot, fry the pepper on each side for 6 to 8 minutes. Take the pepper out of the oven. Let it cool down a bit, remove the hard skin.
3. Chopped jalapeno very fine. If you don't like heat, remove seeds before chopping. You can also start with 1 teaspoon of jalapeno before adding the second teaspoon. Finely chop the Poblano pepper.
4. Add chopped coriander, salt, bell pepper and red onions. Mix in the lemon juice and lime juice. Mix the salsa well. Place in the refrigerator for a few hours before serving. This allows the flavors to marry together.

Nutrition 34 Calories 1g Protein 8g Fat

Tzatziki sauce

Preparation time: 21 minutes

Cooking time: 33 minutes

Servings: 4

Ingredients

- 2 natural yogurts
- 1 cucumber
- 1 clove garlic
- 4 fresh mint leaves
- 1 teaspoon dill
- Lemon juice c / n
- Salt and ground black pepper c / n

Direction

1. To make the Greek cucumber and yogurt sauce, peel the cucumber and open it in half.
2. Remove the seeds, grate it and let it drain in a colander with a little salt to remove excess water. Squeeze occasionally with a spoon to speed up this process.
3. Dry between absorbent paper and put it in a bowl. Drain the yogurts in a colander and add it to the bowl.
4. Add the peeled and crushed garlic clove, dill, chopped peppermint leaves, salt, ground black pepper to taste and a few drops of lemon juice.
5. Mix the ingredients very well to obtain a tzatziki sauce, test and rectify if necessary. Let stand in the fridge for 30 minutes and serve cold with vegetables or pieces of bread to spread or accompany beef, poultry or fish.

Nutrition 391 calories 21g fat 18g protein

Homemade Pesto

Preparation time: 55 minutes

Cooking time: 15 minutes

Servings: 4

Ingredients:

- 100 gr of basil leaves
- 200 gr of Parmesan cheese
- 75 gr of pine nuts
- 2 cloves of garlic
- 160 ml olive oil
- Salt

Direction

1. We prepare the main ingredient of this homemade pesto recipe, basil. You have to separate the leaves of the stem well. This step is important because the stem tends to slightly bitter the taste of the dish.

2. Next, we will wash and dry the basil well. We can put it on absorbent paper so that it leaves all the water that may have fallen. Otherwise, if any trace remains, it may cause it to rust and change the color and taste of the dish. It will darken shortly and stop having that intense green color so characteristic.

3. Peel the garlic cloves and cut them into small pieces. We begin to prepare the pine nuts in a pan, sauté them without oil to acquire that peculiar roasted flavor.

4. In the blender glass, we will place the cloves of garlic, pine nuts, basil, and cheese, with a little olive oil. We

crush it very well and start creating the most traditional pesto. The texture and taste are unmistakable. Prepare homemade pasta and enjoy a really exciting dish.

Nutrition 407 Calories 7g Protein 42g Fat

Hollandaise Sauce

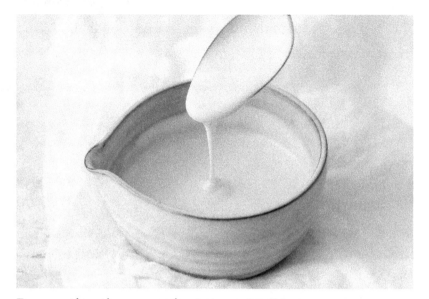

Preparation time: 14 minutes

Cooking time: 9 minutes

Servings: 4

Ingredient

- 200 gr. of butter
- 4 egg yolks
- Juice of 1/2 lemon or 1 tablespoon of white wine
- A pinch of salt

Directions:

1. Melt the butter in a saucepan by removing the foam that appears on the surface, and let it temper.
2. Put the egg yolks in a bowl and beat them with a rod blender. When they begin to assemble, add the melted butter little by little, being careful not to add the serum

that is left in the bottom, while stirring until you get a fine cream.

3. Add the juice of 1/2 lemon or a tablespoon of white wine and a pinch of salt while stirring. Serve the hollandaise sauce.

Nutrition 247 Calories 2g Protein 26g Fat

Red Pesto

Preparation time: 55 minutes

Cooking time: 15 minutes

Servings: 4

Ingredients:

- 50g grated Parmesan cheese
- 100c.c. Of olive oil
- 10 dried tomatoes
- 10 fresh basil leaves
- 1 tablespoon pine nuts
- 1 clove garlic

Directions

1. Place the dried tomatoes in a bowl and let them soak for at least 20 minutes. Drain and reserve.
2. Put a pan on the fire without oil or butter and place them, stir occasionally so they do not burn.
3. Place the dried tomatoes in the blender glass and add the roasted pine nuts, washed basil leaves, peeled and chopped garlic clove, grated Parmesan cheese, and olive oil.
4. Crush all the ingredients until you get a thick red pesto sauce.
5. Store the red pesto in a previously sterilized glass jar. Close it very well and keep it in the fridge for up to 7 days.

Nutrition: 716 Calories 9g Protein 7g Fat

Keto Pesto Sauce with Parmesan

Preparation time: 11 minutes

Cooking time: 32 minutes

Servings: 4

Ingredient

- 60 gr fresh basil leaves
- 35 g lightly toasted pine nuts
- 2 pcs. cloves of garlic
- 30 gr extra virgin olive oil
- 25 gr grated Parmesan cheese
- 12 pinches of salt
- 13 table. spoon. pure water

Direction

1. Lightly brown the pine nuts until golden brown in a dry skillet over medium heat. Transfer to another dish and let cool.

2. In a food processor or blender, combine basil leaves, pine nuts, garlic, olive oil and Parmesan cheese. Mix for a few minutes until a smooth paste is formed. It is best not to grind the sauce into a smooth paste, but leave the texture of the food.

3. Add salt to taste. If the sauce is thick, add a little water and stir.

Nutrition 155 Calories 13g Fat 18g Protein

Keto Pesto Sauce

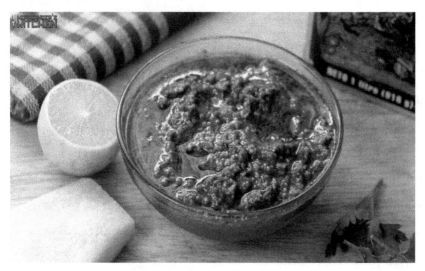

Preparation time: 21 minutes

Cooking time: 33 minutes

Servings: 6

Ingredient

- 2 cups freshly chopped basil
- 4 pcs. cloves of garlic
- 1/3 glass of pine nuts
- 2/3 glass of grated Parmesan cheese
- ½ cup unrefined olive oil
- 1 tea spoon. salt
- 1 tea spoon. pepper

Direction

1. In a deep bowl, combine the basil, garlic, pine nuts, and parmesan cheese. Grind with a blender until smooth.
2. Gradually add olive oil as you mix.

3. Add salt and pepper at the end, stir again. The pesto sauce is ready.

Nutrition 173 Calories 14g Fat 7g Protein

Keto Sauce Béchamel with Cream Cheese

Preparation time: 11 minutes

Cooking time: 0 minutes

Servings: 6

Ingredient

- 2 cups heavy whipping cream
- 200 gr creamy soft cheese
- ½ tea spoon. salt
- ¼ tea. spoon. ground black pepper
- ¼ tea. spoon. nutmeg

Direction

1. Add all ingredients to a non-stick saucepan or skillet and stir.
2. Place the saucepan over medium heat. Bring to a boil, stirring constantly.
3. Reduce heat and simmer for a few minutes until the sauce thickens. Make sure that the mass does not burn.

Nutrition 351 Calories 36g Fat 4g Protein

Creamy Keto Sauce with Lemon Pepper

Preparation time: 22 minutes

Cooking time: 8 minutes

Servings: 6

Ingredient

- cups heavy whipping cream
- 1 cup a mixture of shredded Parmesan, Provolone, Asiago
- 2 tea. spoon. lemon pepper

Direction

1. Combine all ingredients in a nonstick saucepan or skillet.
2. Simmer over low heat for about 20 minutes, stirring occasionally. When the sauce has thickened, you can remove it from the stove.
3. Serve hot or pour into a lidded container and refrigerate.

Nutrition 284 Calories 28g Fat 5.9g Protein

PASTA RECIPES

Three Cheese Chicken Penne from Applebee's

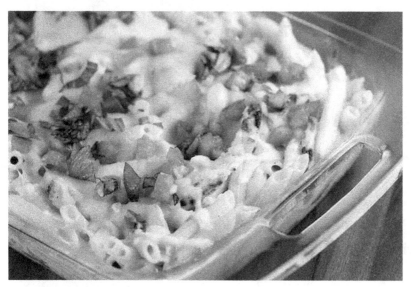

Preparation Time: 10 minutes

Cooking Time: 1 hour

Servings: 4

Ingredients:

- 2 boneless skinless chicken breasts
- 1 cup Italian salad dressing
- 3 cups penne pasta
- 6 tablespoons olive oil, divided
- 15 ounces Alfredo sauce

- 8 ounces combination mozzarella, Parmesan, and provolone cheeses, grated
- 4 roma tomatoes, seeded and diced
- 4 tablespoons fresh basil, diced
- 2 cloves garlic, finely chopped
- Shredded parmesan cheese for serving

Directions:

1. Preheat oven to 350°F.
2. In a bowl, add chicken then drizzle with Italian dressing. Mix to fully coat chicken with dressing. Cover using plastic wrap and keep inside refrigerator overnight but, if you're in a hurry, at least 2 hours is fine.
3. Follow instructions on package to cook penne pasta. Drain, then set aside.
4. Brush 3 tablespoons oil onto grates of grill then preheat to medium-high heat. Add marinated chicken onto grill, discarding the marinade. Cook chicken until both sides are fully cooked and internal temperature measures 165°F. Remove from grill. Set aside until cool enough to handle. Then, cut chicken into thin slices.
5. In a large bowl, add cooked noodles, Alfredo sauce, and grilled chicken. Mix until combined.
6. Drizzle remaining oil onto large casserole pan, then pour noodle mixture inside. Sprinkle cheeses on top. Bake for about 15-20 minutes or until cheese turns a golden and edges of mixture begins to bubble. Remove from oven.
7. Mix tomatoes, basil, and garlic in a bowl. Add on top of pasta.

8. Sprinkle parmesan cheese before serving.

Nutrition: Calories 1402, Total fat 93 g, Saturated fat 27 g, Carbs 91 g,

Sugar 7 g, Fibers 3 g, Protein 62 g, Sodium 5706 mg

Macaroni Grill's Pasta Milano

Preparation Time: 5 minutes

Cooking Time: 20 minutes

Servings: 6

Ingredients:

- 1 pound bowtie pasta
- 2 teaspoons olive oil
- 1 pound chicken, chopped into small pieces
- 1 12-ounce package mushrooms, chopped
- 1 cup onion, minced
- 2 garlic cloves, finely minced
- 1/2 cup sun dried tomatoes, diced
- 1 1/2 cups half and half
- 1 tablespoon butter, softened
- 1/2 cup Parmesan cheese, shredded, plus some more for serving
- 1 teaspoon black pepper, ground
- 1 tablespoon fresh basil, minced

Directions:

1. Follow instructions on package to cook bowtie pasta. Drain, then set aside.
2. Add oil to a pan over medium-high heat. Once hot, add chicken and stir-fry for about 5 to 6 minutes until cooked through. Set chicken aside onto a plate.
3. In the same pan, toss in mushrooms, onions, garlic, and sun-dried tomatoes. Sauté until onions turn soft and

mushrooms become a light brown, then sprinkle salt and pepper to season. Return chicken to pan and mix.

4. Mix half and half, butter, Parmesan, pepper, and basil in a small bowl.

5. Add half and half mixture to pan. Stir, and let simmer for about 3 to 4 minutes or until pan ingredients are thoroughly heated. Mix in pasta until coated well.

6. Serve.

Nutrition: Calories 600, Total fat 18 g, Saturated fat 9 g, Carbs 69 g,
Sugar 8 g, Fibers 5 g, Protein 42 g, Sodium 349 mg

Olive Garden's Fettuccine Alfredo

Preparation Time: 5 minutes

Cooking Time: 25 minutes

Servings: 6

Ingredients:

- 1/2 cup butter, melted
- 2 tablespoons cream cheese
- 1-pint heavy cream
- 1 teaspoon garlic powder
- Some salt
- Some black pepper
- 2/3 cup parmesan cheese, grated
- 1 pound fettuccine, cooked

Directions:

1. Melt the cream cheese in the melted butter over medium heat until soft.
2. Add the heavy cream and season the mixture with garlic powder, salt, and pepper.
3. Reduce the heat to low and allow the mixture to simmer for another 15 to 20 minutes.
4. Remove the mixture from heat and add in the parmesan. Stir everything to melt the cheese.
5. Pour the sauce over the pasta and serve.

Nutrition: Calories: 767.3 Fat: 52.9 g Carbs: 57.4 g Protein: 17.2 g

Sodium: 367 mg

Red Lobster's Shrimp Pasta

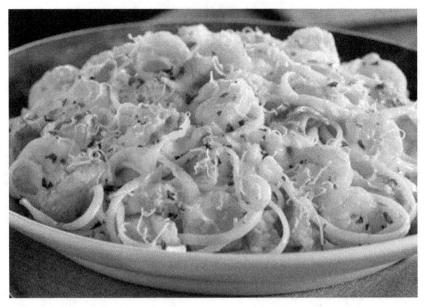

Preparation Time: 5 minutes

Cooking Time: 30 minutes

Servings: 4

Ingredients:

- 8 ounces linguini or spaghetti pasta
- 1/3 cup extra virgin olive oil
- 3 garlic cloves
- 1 pound shrimp, peeled, deveined
- 2/3 cup clam juice or chicken broth
- 1/3 cup white wine
- 1 cup heavy cream
- 1/2 cup parmesan cheese, freshly grated
- 1/4 teaspoon dried basil, crushed
- 1/4 teaspoon dried oregano, crushed

- Fresh parsley and parmesan cheese for garnish

Directions:

1. Cook the Pasta according to package directions. Simmer the garlic in hot oil over low heat, until tender. Increase the heat to low to medium and add the shrimp. When the shrimp is

2. Cooked, transfer it to a separate bowl along with the garlic. Keep the remaining oil in the pan. Pour the clam or chicken broth into the pan and bring to a boil.

3. Add the wine and adjust the heat to medium. Keep cooking the mixture for another 3 minutes. While stirring the mixture, reduce the heat to low and add in the cream and cheese. Keep stirring. When the mixture thickens, return the shrimp to the pan and throw in the remaining ingredients (except the pasta). Place the pasta in a bowl and pour the sauce over it. Mix everything together and serve. Garnish with parsley and parmesan cheese, if desired

Nutrition: Calories: 590 Fat: 26 g Carbs: 54 g Protein: 34 g Sodium: 1500 mg

Olive Garden's Steak Gorgonzola

Preparation Time: 10 minutes

Cooking Time: 1 hour and 30 minutes

Servings: 6

Ingredients:

Pasta:

- 1/2 pounds boneless beef top sirloin steaks, cut into 1/2-inch cubes
- 1 pound fettucine or linguini, cooked
- 2 tablespoons sun-dried tomatoes, chopped
- 2 tablespoons balsamic vinegar glaze
- Some fresh parsley leaves, chopped

Marinade:

- 1/2 cups Italian dressing
- 1 tablespoon fresh rosemary, chopped
- 1 tablespoon fresh lemon juice (optional)
- Spinach Gorgonzola Sauce:
- 4 cups baby spinach, trimmed
- 2 cups Alfredo sauce (recipe follows)
- 1/2 cup green onion, chopped
- 6 tablespoons gorgonzola, crumbled, and divided)

Directions:

1. Cook the pasta and set aside. Mix together the marinade ingredients in a
2. Sealable container.
3. Marinate the beef in the container for an hour.

4. While the beef is marinating, make the Spinach Gorgonzola sauce. Heat the Alfredo sauce in a saucepan over medium heat. Add spinach and green onions. Let simmer until the spinach wilt. Crumble 4 tablespoons of the Gorgonzola cheese on top of the sauce. Let melt and stir. Set aside remaining 2 tablespoons of the cheese for garnish. Set aside and cover with lid to keep warm.

5. When the beef is done marinating, grill each piece depending on your preference.

6. Toss the cooked pasta and the Alfredo sauce in a saucepan, and then transfer to a plate.

7. Top the pasta with the beef, and garnish with balsamic glaze, sun-dried tomatoes, crumble gorgonzola cheese, and parsley leaves.

8. Serve and enjoy.

Nutrition: Calories: 740.5 Fat: 27.7 g Carbs: 66 g Protein: 54.3 g Sodium: 848.1 mg

DESSERT RECIPES

Cheesecake Factory's White Chocolate Raspberry Truffle Cheesecake

Preparation Time: 2 h + overnight refrigeration

Cooking Time: 1 h 12 min

Servings: 24

Ingredients:

- Oreo Crust
- 1 1/2 cups Oreo baking crumbs
- 1/3 cup butter, melted
- Raspberry Sauce
- 10 ounces fresh raspberries, washed, rinsed and dried with paper towels
- 1/4 cup sugar
- 2 tablespoons lemon juice

Filling

- 4 (8-ounce) packs cream cheese, at room temperature
- 1 1/4 cups sugar
- 1/2 cup sour cream, at room temperature
- 2 teaspoons vanilla
- 5 eggs, at room temperature
- 4 ounces white chocolate, chopped
- Garnish

- 1 cup heavy whipping cream
- 1/2 cup powdered sugar
- White chocolate shavings, for garnish

Directions:

1. Preheat oven to 475°F. Line a spring form pan. Wrap the outer part of the pan with aluminum foil as well.

2. Place a large pan filled 1/2-inch deep with water in the oven as it heats. Make sure to maintain the water at this level.

3. Combine the crumbs and butter well and press into the bottom of the spring form pan. Cover and freeze until filling is ready.

4. To make the raspberry sauce, combine the ingredients in a saucepan and bring to a boil. With constant stirring, simmer until raspberries are broken down. Strain into a mixing bowl and let cool. Set aside.

5. Place cream cheese, sugar, sour cream and vanilla in a bowl for an electric mixer. Set speed to low and mix until smooth.

6. Add eggs one at a time, while mixing, until well-blended.

7. Sprinkle the bottom of the crust with the chopped white chocolate.

8. Pour half of the filling into the pan, spreading with a spatula.

9. Scoop out about 1/3 cup of the cooled raspberry sauce and store any remaining sauce for future recipes.

10. Pour half of the scooped raspberry sauce into the filling and then make a quick swirl with a butter knife.

11. Add the rest of the filling and swirl in the remaining raspberry sauce.
12. Place the pan (with outer bottom lined) in the water bath.
13. Bake for 12 minutes, then reduce oven temperature to 350°F.
14. Continue baking until top of cheesecake turns light brown (about 1 hour).
15. Do not open the oven. Leave the pan in the oven to cool completely (about 1-2 hours).
16. Remove from oven, cover with plastic wrap and refrigerate overnight.
17. Whip the cream and powdered sugar rapidly (about 5 minutes).
18. Remove cheesecake from pan and sprinkle with white chocolate shavings.
19. Serve with whipped cream.

Nutrition: Calories 365, Total Fat 25 g, Carbs 31 g, Protein 5 g, Sodium 199 mg

Buca Di Beppo's Italian Crème Cake

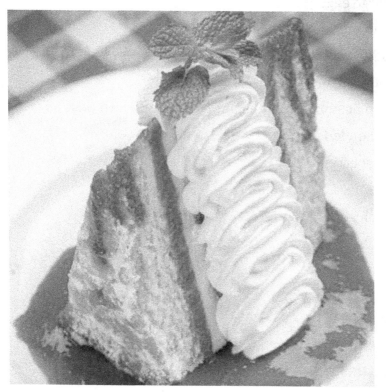

Preparation Time: 40 min

Cooking Time: 30 min

Servings: 8-12

Ingredients:

Cake

- 2 cups all-purpose flour
- 2 teaspoons baking powder
- 1/2 teaspoon salt
- Juice and zest of 1 medium lemon
- 1/2 cup unsalted butter, softened

- 1 1/4 cups granulated sugar
- 3 large eggs
- 1 cup milk

Filling and Frosting

- 8 ounces mascarpone, softened
- 1 cup heavy cream, plus more for garnish (if desired)
- 1/2 cup lemon curd
- Raspberry Sauce
- 12 ounces fresh raspberries
- 1 tablespoon sugar
- 1 tablespoon brandy (optional)

Directions:

1. Preheat oven to 350°F. Line and butter two 9-inch round pans.
2. In a bowl, combine flour, baking powder, salt, and lemon zest, then set aside.
3. Using an electric mixer, cream the butter and sugar until light and fluffy.
4. Keeping speed at medium, add eggs one at a time, mixing well after each addition.
5. Mix in the lemon juice and reduce speed to low.
6. Add dry ingredients and milk alternately until well-blended.
7. Pour equal amounts into prepared pans and spread evenly.
8. Bake until a toothpick inserted into the center of the cakes comes out clean (about 30 minutes).
9. Cool the cakes in the pans for 10 minutes.

10. Remove from pans and let cool completely on a wire rack.
11. While the cakes are cooling, prepare the frosting/filling. Mix the ingredients until smooth. If needed, cover with plastic wrap and keep refrigerated while waiting for cakes to cool completely.
12. To prepare the raspberry sauce, mix the ingredients using a food processor or blender. Cover and refrigerate until ready to use.
13. If needed, slice off any uneven parts of the tops of the cakes. Spread with frosting and place one on top of the other.
14. Pipe whipped cream over frosting, if desired, and drizzle with raspberry sauce.

Nutrition: Calories 765, Total Fat 42 g, Carbs 93 g, Protein 8 g, Sodium 337 mg

Corner Bakery Café's Cinnamon Crème Coffee Cake

Preparation Time: 30 min

Cooking Time: 1 h 15 min

Servings: 8-12

Ingredients:

- Filling and Streusel
- 1/2 cup sugar
- 2/3 Cup brown sugar
- 1 tablespoon cinnamon
- 1/4 teaspoon nutmeg
- 22/3 cups flour
- 1 cup (2 sticks) butter, melted
- Cake
- 3 cups flour
- 2 teaspoons baking powder
- 1 teaspoon baking soda
- 1/4 teaspoon salt
- 1/2 cup (1 stick) butter, diced, at room temperature
- 1/2 cup vegetable shortening
- 1 1/2 cups sugar
- 5 eggs
- 1 1/2 teaspoons vanilla
- 2 cups sour cream
- Powdered sugar, for dusting

Directions:

1. Preheat oven to 350°F. Grease and flour a tube pan.
2. First prepare the streusel. In a bowl, mix together sugars, cinnamon, nutmeg and flour.
3. Add the melted butter and mix to form large morsels (do not break into fine crumbs).
4. Now prepare the cake batter. Combine flour, baking powder, baking soda and salt. Set aside.
5. In a large bowl, place the butter and shortening.
6. Add sugar and beat until light and creamy.
7. Beat in vanilla.
8. Gradually add the flour mixture and sour cream, alternately, to make a thick batter.
9. Put half of the batter into the tube pan and put half of the streusel over it.
10. Add the remaining batter and top with the remaining streusel, gently pressing down to set into the batter.
11. Bake until toothpick inserted near center comes out clean (about 1 hour 15 minutes).
12. Let cool for 30 minutes.
13. Remove from pan and let cool on a wire rack.
14. Dust with powdered sugar.

Nutrition: Calories 780, Total Fat 37 g, Carbs 104 g, Protein 0.8 g, Sodium 790 mg

Starbucks' Raspberry Swirl Pound Cake

Preparation Time: 20 min

Cooking Time: 55-60 min

Servings: 8

Ingredients:

- 1 box pound cake mix
- 1/4 cup (1/2 stick) butter, at room temperature
- 2 eggs
- 2/3 cup milk
- 1 teaspoon lemon juice
- 1/3 cup raspberry spread
- 6 drops red food color (optional)
- Cream Cheese Frosting
- 1 (8-ounce) package cream cheese, at room temperature
- 1 cup powdered sugar
- 1 teaspoon lemon juice

Directions:

1. Preheat oven to 350°F. Grease and flour a loaf pan.
2. Mix cake mix, milk, butter and eggs with an electric mixer, at low speed, until blended (about 30 seconds). Switch speed to medium and mix 2 minutes more.
3. Pour about 1/3 of the batter into a separate bowl, for the raspberry swirl.
4. To the original bowl, mix in lemon juice.
5. To the other bowl, mix in raspberry spread and food color (if using).
6. Pour about 1/2 of the white batter into the loaf pan.

7. Pour about 1/2 of the raspberry batter on top.

8. Repeat layering red and white layers.

9. Cut through the batter with a spatula, lengthwise, to create the swirl.

10. Bake until just a few crumbs stick to a toothpick inserted at the center (about 55-60 minutes).

11. Place on a wire rack to cool completely.

12. Meanwhile, prepare the cream cheese frosting. Cream the cheese using a mixer until fluffy. Mix in powdered sugar to incorporate. Add lemon juice and mix at low speed until smooth.

13. Frost cooled loaf and serve.

Nutrition: Calories 420, Total Fat 17 g, Carbs 61 g, Protein 6 g,

Sodium 280 mg

The Cheesecake Factory's Copycat Ultimate Red Velvet Cheesecake

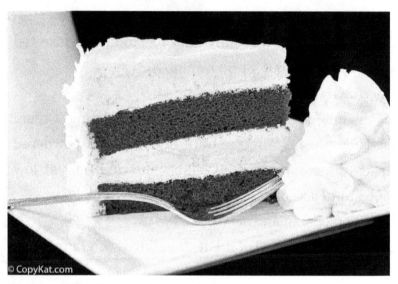

Preparation Time: 3 h 30 min

Cooking Time: 1 h 15 min

Servings: 16

Ingredients:

Cheesecake:

- 2 8-ounce packages cream cheese, softened
- 2/3 cup granulated white sugar
- 1 pinch salt
- 2 large eggs
- 1/3 cup sour cream
- 1/3 cup heavy whipping cream
- 1 teaspoon vanilla extract
- Non-stick cooking spray
- Hot water, for water bath

Red velvet cake:

- 2 1/2 cups all-purpose flour
- 1 1/2 cups granulated white sugar
- 3 tablespoons unsweetened cocoa powder
- 1 1/2 teaspoons baking soda
- 1 teaspoon salt
- 2 large eggs
- 1 1/2 cups vegetable oil
- 1 cup buttermilk
- 1/4 cup red food coloring
- 2 teaspoons vanilla extract
- 2 teaspoons white vinegar

Frosting:

- 2 1/2 cups powdered sugar, sifted
- 2 8-ounce packages cream cheese, softened
- 1/2 cup unsalted butter, softened
- 1 tablespoon vanilla extract

Directions:

1. For the cheesecake, preheat oven to 325°F.
2. Mix cream cheese, sugar, and salt using a mixer for about 2 minutes until creamy and smooth. Add eggs, mixing again after adding each one. Add sour cream, heavy cream, and vanilla extract until smooth and well blended.
3. Coat spring form pan with non-stick cooking spray, then place parchment paper on top. Wrap outsides of Spring

Form pan entirely with two layers of aluminum foil. This is preventing water bath from entering the pan.

4. Pour cream cheese batter into Spring Form pan, then place into a roasting pan. Add boiling water to roasting pan to surround Spring Form pan. Place in oven and bake for 45 minutes until set.

5. Transfer Spring Form pan with cheesecake onto a rack to cool for about 1 hour. Freeze overnight.

6. For the red velvet cake, preheat oven to 350°F.

7. Combine flour, sugar, cocoa powder, baking soda, and salt in a large bowl. In a separate bowl, mix eggs, oil, buttermilk, food coloring, vanilla and vinegar. Add wet ingredients to dry ingredients. Blend for 1 minute with a mixer on medium-low speed, then on high speed for 2 minutes.

8. Spray non-stick cooking spray to 2 metal baking pans that are the same size as the Spring Form pan earlier. Coat bottoms thinly with flour. Then, pour equal amounts cake batter onto bottom of pans.

9. Place in oven and bake for about 30 to 35 minutes. Cake is done once only a few crumbs attach to a toothpick when inserted. Transfer to a rack and let cool for 10 minutes. Separate cake from pan using a knife on the edges, then invert onto rack. Let cool.

10. To prepare frosting, mix powdered sugar, cream cheese, butter, and vanilla using a mixer on medium-high speed just enough until smooth.

11. Assemble cake by positioning 1st red velvet cake layer onto a cake plate. Remove cheesecake from pan, remove parchment paper, and layer on top of red velvet cake layer. Then, top with 2nd red velvet cake layer.

12. Coat a thin layer of prepared frosting onto entire outside of cake. Clean spatula every time you scoop out from bowl of frosting so as to not mix crumbs into it. Refrigerate for 30 minutes to set. Then, coat cake with 2nd layer by adding a large scoop on top then spreading it to the top side of the cake then around it.

13. Cut into slices. Serve.

Nutrition: Calories 722, Total Fat 51 g, Carbs 64 g, Protein 9 g,
Sodium 460 mg

Keto Copycat Lemon Bread from Starbucks

Preparation Time: 13 minutes

Cooking Time: 45 minutes

Serving: 15

Ingredients:

- Eggs – 6
- Salt – ½ tsp.
- Zest of 2 lemons (keep one tsp. for glaze)
- Vanilla – 1 tsp.
- Cream cheese (not chilled) – 2 tbsp.
- Monk fruit Classic – 2/3 cup
- Baking powder – 1 ½ tsp.
- Heavy whipping cream 2 tbsp.
- Butter – 9 tbsp.
- Coconut flour – ½ cup and 2 tbsp.
- Fresh lemon juice – 4 tsp.

For glaze:

- Monk fruit powder – 2 tbsp.
- Heavy whipping cream – 1 splash
- Freshly squeezed lemon juice – 2 tsp.
- Lemon zest – 1 tsp.

Direction:

1. To attain 325 degrees Fahrenheit, warm the oven. Using a sheet of parchment baking paper, prepare a bread pan.

2. To melt the butter, add it to a microwaveable bowl. Just let it cool.
3. Whisk together the eggs, heavy whipping cream, vanilla, monk fruit classic, baking powder, cream cheese and salt until mixed.
4. Mix the coconut flour, lemon zest, melted butter, and juice thoroughly with the mixture.
5. Pour the batter into the bread pan that has been prepared.
6. Bake it until it only begins to get brown on the top of the bread, and a toothpick inserted in the middle comes out clean (55 minutes to one hour).
7. By blending the lemon juice with lemon zest, monk fruit powder, and a splash of heavy whipping cream, prepare the glaze. Whisk until it's creamy.
8. Put the prepared glaze over the hot bread, lay it out in such a way that the top is covered and dripped on the sides. Serve and enjoy.

Nutrition 121 Calories 5g Fat 11g Protein

Keto Copycat Strawberries Romanoff from La Madeleine

Preparation Time: 14 minutes
Cooking Time: 7 minutes
Serving: 4
Ingredients:

- Strawberries – 1 pound or 2 pints
- Artificial sweetener – 2 tbsp.
- Heavy cream – 1 cup
- Brandy – 4 tbsp.

Direction

1. Rinse the strawberries and cut off their tops. Let them get drained.
2. Mix the artificial sweetener, heavy whipping cream, and the brandy together. Beat it with the help of a mixer until it gets dense or thick.
3. Put the strawberries in the glasses and put the sauce on top with a spoon. Prepare 3 to 4 servings and enjoy.

Nutrition 303 Calories 21g Protein 9g Fat

Keto Copycat Brownies from KFC

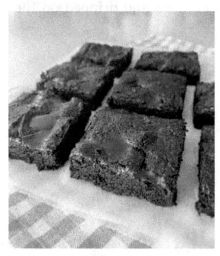

Preparation Time: 13 minutes
Cooking Time: 45 minutes

Serving: 16

Ingredients:

- Butter – ½ cup
- Almond flour – ½ cup
- Baking powder – ¼ tsp.
- Vanilla – 1 tsp.
- Eggs – 2
- Salt – ¼ tsp.
- Artificial sweetener – 1 cup
- Cocoa powder (Hershey's) – 1/3 cup
- Optional: Walnuts (broken into pieces) – ¼ cup

Direction:

1. Preheat the oven to 350 degrees Fahrenheit.
2. Line with foil and butter the foil in an 8-inch square tray.
3. Sift the cocoa, almond flour, salt, and baking powder together. Melt butter over low heat in a saucepan of ten to twelve cups of capacity. Stir in the butter the vanilla, and artificial sweetener.
4. Enable the warm mixture to cool down for five minutes, then remove the pan from the burner. Stir in the eggs immediately, so they won't cook because of heat. (Before adding in the eggs, it is best to break all of the eggs in a bowl.)
5. Add the dry ingredients, and stir in the nuts. Spread in the prepared pan smoothly. Bake for 20 to 25 minutes.
6. Cool for 15 minutes. Cover with a rack and switch around the pan. Remove the lining of the pan and foil. Cover and

switch back over again with a cutting board. Let it stand till it's cool.

Nutrition 174 Calories 13g Fat 9g Protein

Keto Copycat Lemon Lush from Drummer's Cafe

Preparation Time: 13 minutes

Cooking Time: 45 minutes

Serving: 24

Ingredients

For the crust:

- Chopped nuts (low carb nuts) – ½ cup
- Butter – 4 oz.
- Almond flour – 1 cup

For the lemon layer:

- Almond milk – 3 cups
- Instant pudding mix – 2 packages
- For the creamy top layer:
- Erythritol – 1 cup
- Cream cheese – 8 oz.
- Cool whip – 1 cup

Direction

1. Mix the melted butter, almond flour, and chopped nuts together. Spread into a tray that is 9x13" in size. Bake for 15 minutes at 350 degrees. Prior to pouring the pudding on top, cool the crust for 15 minutes.

2. Mix the pudding and milk together. Beat until thickening begins. Pour this over the nut crust that has been cooled.

3. Mix the cream cheese, cool whip, and erythritol together and scatter over the lemon pudding.

Nutrition 172 Calories 14g Fat 11g Protein

Keto Copycat Fat Bombs from Karibu Cafe

Preparation Time: 11 minutes

Cooking Time: 5 minutes

Serving: 10

Ingredients:

- Grass-fed butter – ¼ cup
- Powdered erythritol – ¼ cup
- Coffee extract – ½ tsp.
- Organic coconut oil – ¼ cup
- Mascarpone cheese (at room temperature) – ¼ cup
- Dark chocolate (sugar-free) – 1 bar
- Unsweetened cocoa powder – 2tbsp.

Direction:

1. Using a hand mixer or whisk, add the mascarpone cheese, butter, and coconut oil to a bowl.
2. Add the erythritol, cocoa powder, coffee extract powder and mix until well mixed together.
3. Add to the silicone liners (mini muffins one) or ice cube trays and add chopped chocolate on top. With your fingertips, press the chocolate down softly. To set, freeze for 20 minutes. Keep it in the refrigerator or freezer.

Nutrition 116 Calories 1g Fat 3g Protein

CONCLUSION

You reached this part of the book, then I must congratulate you, as you have unlocked all the culinary secrets behind the irresistible restaurant like flavorsome meals.

No matter how many times we visit these restaurants, there is always a part of us that keeps wanting those amazing flavors a little bit more. Instead of spending so much on the dining out, it is super smart to recreate those same meals at home.

And you already love cooking, then this cookbook will excite you to the core, as it has brought together all the delicious and fancy meals from the world-renowned restaurants in one place. The restaurants listed in this cookbook, undoubtedly, have no parallel in terms of taste and quality of food. And no other restaurant can replace their fine flavors. With all the recipes shared in this cookbook, now you can carry their menu with you and recreate their super delicious menu anywhere at any time.

These recipes can serve all your food needs quite well; whether it's your routine meals or a fancy one for a special occasion, you can cook with healthy and organic ingredients to bring good flavors and lots of nutrients to your dinner tables.

Copycat Recipes can be prepared through their secret recipes. All these recipes have been independently developed and sourced by the respective restaurant's individual home economist and research team.

When cooking copycat recipes, you will be aiming to reproduce the same textures, tastes, and mouthwatering flavors alike. There is nothing more inspiring than a delicious home cooked meal from the restaurant of your choice creating that same satiates with amazing flavors you relish every day. Scroll down through these amazing copycat recipes and see if there's anything that strikes your fancy. Your cooking skills will be a lot more flavorful and delightful when you cook using these recipes at home. Start cooking and have fun!

CPSIA information can be obtained
at www.ICGtesting.com
Printed in the USA
BVHW062328220321
603180BV00003B/437

9 781801 830331